Fres D. Jacobo CNA/HHA

How to be a Successful Caregiver

Turning Your Passion For Caring into a Successful Business

How To Be A Successful Caregiver

How to be a Successful Caregiver

Turning Your Passion For Caring into a Successful Business

by

Fres D. Jacobo, C.N.A./H.H.A.

How To Be A Successful Caregiver
Turning your passion for caring into a successful business
By Fres D. Jacobo

Written by Maria Fres Jacobo and John Paul Ouvrier

Published by JohnPaul Ouvrier

"This book does not constitute medical advice in anyway. Before taking any advice herein, please refer to the medical staff and family in charge of the person. Any followed advice, whether directly or implied that is followed is the sole responsibility of the reader, no matter what their position. We do not take any responsibility in anyway, for anyone, for any reason. If this is a problem, please return this book to the publisher above for a full refund."

More information, such as appendixes, referral sources, etc, will be available in future additions. Please send any ideas and/or material to Fres or John directly. HowToBeASuccessfulCaregiver.Com

First Edition 2014/2015 ~W.A.G.B.Y.H~ I.L.Y.S.M.P.P.G.~Y.D.B.~

Contact information: Fresjacobo@outlook.com

Dedication:

To God who has given me life. Thank you.

To My Sons Marton and Donn Marc.
You have made me a proud mother, Mahal Ko Kayo.

To all my lovely patients:

Thank you for your trust, love, and care.
I am honored to have served you.

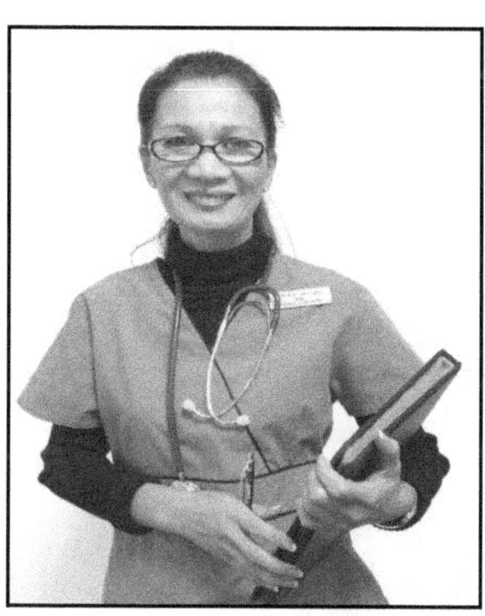

Biography

Biography

Fres D. Jacobo has been a licensed caregiver for over 25 years. One of the most popular and in demand caregivers in the industry, Fres is an inspiration to everyone she meets.

In the 1980s, Fres emigrated to the United States of America from the Philippines. Through hard work and patience, she was later able to bring her children to the United States and help them become citizens. They have each gone to college and are successful in their own right.

Please join with Fres as she shares with you her journey and the business secrets she learned along the way. May her story inspire and bless you, and may you share these gifts with others.

You may reach Fres via email at:
FresJacobo@outlook.com

Table of Contents

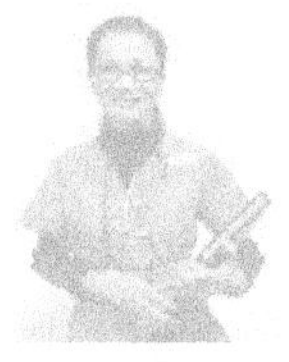

INTRODUCTION

Would you like to be a **Successful Caregiver**? You can be. Would you like to learn the skills that are not taught in school that all successful caregivers practice? Would you like to be the person with those skills that families, individuals, and agencies want to hire first? Then this book is for you.

This is the best time in history to enter into the lucrative world of professional caregiving. Never before has an older population that needs assistance existed. And while this book is designed to address the professional caregiver within the United States, the principles are for everyone to use, no matter which country you live in. (Therefore, when I refer to the United States, or Americans, please substitute whichever country you will work in if the ideas are appropriate.)

Great things can happen in the caregiving industry; they have happened for me, and they can happen for you. This is an industry that seems simple on the outside, yet requires some careful explaining. Let's get some of the basic misconceptions out of the way:

Successful Caregivers work in ALL areas of society.

There is a myth that holds that caregivers only work for rich people. This is not true. Successful caregivers usually work for older adults who are middle class, and who can afford the services of a caregiver, or their insurance is set up to afford assistance. Most of these seniors live in modest homes or apartments. In order to be hired, you need to understand what they are looking for so that they will want to hire you. We will cover these points within this book.

Successful Caregivers know how to make their services indispensible.

One of the goals of this book is to help you become so good at your job that you become indispensible. This means that your patients enjoy your work so much that they don't want to do without you. Whether you're just starting out after earning your degree, getting ready or going to school, want a career or life change, or already work as a caregiver in its many forms, this book and its rules are designed to show you what the most successful caregivers in the United States (and the world) have in common, thus making your services indispensible. **Successful Caregivers** do not become successful by accident; there are skills to learn and I am honored to share them with you.

It is one of the biggest secrets within the medical industry; **Successful Caregivers** are everywhere! Many caregivers make more than the nurses and medical staff that they work with. And you can do this without compromise or hiding. You can be loved, appreciated, and respected- and drive home in a nice car to go and see your family!

Older patients who seek and employ the services of a caregiver (this could also mean their families or their conservators) have been living in America for some time. More often than not, they know what they will pay for a good person; they pay lots of money for everything else. Don't let anyone convince you take a small paycheck and then work you to death. Don't listen to the abusive person who says you will never find another job. While sometimes in a crisis situation this may be true, those situations are usually temporary though difficult. Please use this book to realize your self-worth and earning potential and don't stop until you get what you want. Now let's cover the basic understandings of the caregiver market here in the United States.

Most Americans (and by American, we mean anyone living in the United States, and they may be of any race or national origin), have a set of unspoken rules that they use to critique you when you work for them.

They will not speak these rules out loud, nor communicate them. They will simply not hire you, or find a way to replace you. In fact many times they may not even be aware of the subtle rule system by which they operate. Add to that Americans are a mix of many cultures and once again, the rules can vary greatly.

This is important to know because if you are not aware of what an older person living in the United States is expecting (consciously or unconsciously), you will not be able to keep them happy, and therefore not keep a steady job or be worried about losing the job you have.

All these ideas can be easily addressed successfully with the ten simple steps in this book. And if for some reason, your patient doesn't like you, you can then be sure it's not about your work ethic or performance.

Throughout this book, you will see "Successful Caregiver Tips" in italics as shown below. These tips are little bits of important information; some of them will pertain to the chapter, others are just common sense. Yet they are important, and should be read. Here is one for you to consider:

***Successful Caregiver Tip**: Understanding your patient's needs means wanting and caring so much that you can see they need help, even before they realize they need help. Successful caregivers know that taking care of another means giving them what they need both mentally and physically before they ask. It means respecting them enough to pay attention to what their needs are, so you can address those needs before they are vocalized. This is a wonderful way to care for your patients.*

Also, at the end of each chapter, I will present a Quick Summary of the main points within that particular chapter so you can easily review and re-read the chapters you are most interested in.

The overall goal of this book is to teach you how to work for yourself, whether that is working for an agency or being self-employed because ultimately you are still working for yourself. The United States loves new businesses in its many forms, and the entire economic system thrives on smaller businesses that connect everyone together in ways that the larger companies cannot. Though each city and state has its own legal issues, starting your own business is not difficult and can be done.

***And as a quick note**: Please pay your taxes. Do not be fooled by others who say to you, that the money you make is, 'under the table.' From a tax liability standpoint, there is no such thing as 'under the table.' All the government sees [in the U.S.A. the tax department of the government is called the I.R.S.] is that when money is collected, taxes are paid.*

Please do what you have to do to get started, but get in the system and start to pay your taxes as soon as you are able. 'Under the table' does not mean tax free, it simply means you responsible for collecting and paying your own taxes. (Please see a qualified tax accountant.)

There are many things to take care of when starting a business. Taking care of these legal issues is beyond the scope of this book. This book is not about getting business permits nor insurance; there are many books written by business people that can help you with this. This book is a carefully crafted series of explanations and understandings on the fundamental business philosophies needed to be a **Successful Caregiver**.

Now let me share with you some definitions that I will refer to within this book. I will address 'us' (the reader and myself) as the 'caregiver'. I will address the people we are taking care of as our 'Boss', or our 'patients', or sometimes 'clients'.

Many caregivers call their patients by different names. Some will say, "My lady or gentleman", or "Mr. or Mrs. Jones", or even "Boss". All these examples are fine as long as they are polite and respectful.

Are you 'Fair', 'Good', or 'Great' at your job? What's your philosophy?

There is a basic law in business that has been true since business began: There are lots of people in any business that are 'fair' and 'good' at their job, yet there are only a few who are great. This book is designed to make you one of the great caregivers that is offered the job first.

Who are these great caregivers? Those that keep quiet and do their job. Those that keep getting the work. Those that the lazy workers complain about. Those that do the little things they don't get paid for. Those that really care, those that really work, those that go out of their way to help others, etc.

Great caregivers don't complain like everyone else; they're too busy working. They don't have time to gossip; they're too busy working. That's a theme you will read about in this book; successful people don't have time to do nothing- they're too busy working! *And the great people are the ones that get and keep the jobs.*

Many outsiders think that the caregiving industry is easy work. And sometimes this industry, like any other industry, attracts people who are in it for the money and they take every short cut possible. They don't do their jobs. They steal from their patients. They ask for money or tell sad stories to get included in their patients will and estates. They don't want to write anything down. They prefer to read and watch TV. They order their patients around. They think the job is like that of a baby sitter who sits and does nothing. Nothing could be further from the truth.

The truth is working in the caregiving industry is one of the hardest jobs in the world. Taking care of a sick and/or elderly patient round the clock requires patience of the highest degree. This patience verges on sainthood in the scheme of things. You will skip meals, lose sleep, have to time your trips to the bathroom around your patient, and the list goes on. There will be days when you understand what Mother Teresa went through.

If any of this scares you, or if you think you can set your business up so you can avoid most of this work, you're wrong. Caregiving is a life dedicated to service. The good news is that if you are willing to give this kind of care to your patients, then there is no reason you shouldn't charge top dollar for this expertise. Giving your best does not mean your best isn't worth a fair wage. What this does mean is that you must give more in service than what you charge.

For instance, charging twenty dollars an hour and giving one hundred dollars an hour in service (work) is fair. Asking twenty dollars an hour and then doing no work is stealing, and that caregiver will lose their job!

Successful Caregiver Tip*: Remember, the best promotional tool in the Caregiver business is the referrals from your existing customers (patients). Who's going to refer a caregiver who sits around all day? Do more than you're paid for each and every day. Soon enough, you will be the one getting the new customers, and one day will have more work than you alone can do...*

Therefore, if you are a person who can save the lives of others, give them a better today and tomorrow, if you want to be needed and important, make a difference, receive fair compensation, and know that you are here for a reason, then this book is for you!

I am honored to be your sister in this journey and humbled to share my years of experience with all of you. God has blessed me in ways I could never have imagined when I was a little girl and a young woman.

I came to this country with only a few dollars in my pocket; now my children are with me and they are United States citizens. And while my goals took me many years to achieve, by the grace of the Lord, I am still here and helping others. I wish for you this success as well.

For what it is worth; I still work. Even as I write these words, I have patients I need to go and see. This book has been a labor of love, and a gift from my heart to your heart.

My words will save you years of work. Yet I know that you will find ways of doing a better job than I have; this is the healthy evolution of any business. You will make yourselves greater than my humble words and deeds have ever made me. And together, we will raise the standards within this industry.

Think about what you would like to happen to you and your family: One day you may have the resources to help your family and loved ones. You could easily have money to send home. You could buy a car or a home. Send your children to school or college. You could find your dreams coming true. *To him that asketh, so shall he receive.*

It is my most sincere wish that you trust your heart, follow your vision and have all your dreams come true. Be proud. You are in one of the greatest careers in the world. It is an honor to be called a caregiver and in so doing, we are all brothers and sisters.

May God grant you many blessings, health, happiness, wealth and love. Thank you so much.

Fres D. Jacobo CNA/HHA
Los Angeles, California, U.S.A.

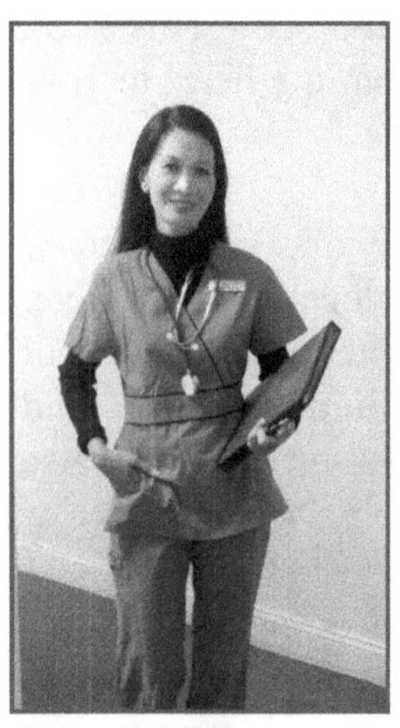

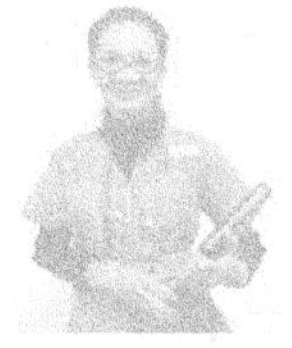

Successful Caregiver Rules Overview:
It's all about RESPECT

There are not enough great caregivers. Let me repeat that; there are not enough great caregivers.

The same is true in every industry. There are never enough great people to do the work that is out there. Every industry is filled with fair to good people. Rare is a great person and the goal of this book is to share the principles that great caregivers share. Great caregivers are always in demand. So your goal, too, should be to become a great caregiver. Let's begin.

The most important word in the caregiver industry is the word RESPECT. Here is how Webster's defines the word respect:

> [1]re·spect ***noun*** \ri-'spekt\ **1:** a relation or reference to a particular thing or situation **2:** an act of giving particular attention: CONSIDERATION **3:** high or special regard: ESTEEM

So let's examine this from a caregiver perspective. Definition one means relating to a particular thing; our patients and those who are working with those patients. Definition two and three are that of 'consideration' and that of 'esteem' toward our patients. In each of these meanings, there is nothing about the caregiver. That is because the job is not about you; it is about the patient.

They say that the way a man looks good is when he does his best to make his woman look good. They say that a great mother is great because she puts her children first. That great is the priest that takes care of his flock. Can you see a pattern here?

When your focus is your patient, you will become great. You will see things that will make your patient comfortable that the other caregivers do not. You will be one step ahead in care and be able to make decisions that will add years to your patients' lives. You will be able to inform the doctors, nurses, and medical staff about things that will make their job easier.

In fact, the medical staff will come to rely on you for up-to-date information about their patient and they will be happy to get it from you. And they will seek this information out because you will give it to them confidently from a pure place in your heart. (We will read about this later.)

***Successful Caregiver Tip**: Referrals can come from a variety of places, but one of the places most caregivers don't consider is the medical professionals they work with. If you help a medical professional do their job and you do a great job in service, they will remember you. And if you remember them as well, their names, something about them, etc, you will be forming a successful professional relationship.*

Sometimes all a medical professional needs is a compliment. And sometimes that professional will be the one to refer you out- so make sure you always have kind word to say, and a business card to hand out. (We will talk about this later as well.)

I have proudly stood and reported to doctors and nurses all the information they needed about their/my patients. I have provided lists and details about what my patients were eating, how they had been sleeping, their mental states, etc.

I have stood assisting doctors and nurses in emergency situations because they had confidence in me and because I gave them critical information. I did not do their job, yet I was able to help them do their job. Because I could help, they wanted my help.

I have been honored to have held the hands of my patients as they were dying. I have been blessed to save the lives of patients dozens of times by doing my job properly; from stopping someone from choking, to calling 911 at the right time, to recognizing something isn't right and taking my patient to the emergency room.

I have seen more love than I knew existed, and I have held back my tears many times. I always say I won't open my heart to my patients, yet I always do. And it is this ability that allows me to give more than I could have ever thought.

So do I think I am great as I write these words? No- I am not. Like you, I wish to be great, and I hope one day I will be, but until then I will do the best I can. I don't think we can do more than this.

If others say I am great, I say, "Thank you so much, now are you going to hire me?" Doing a great job means nothing if it doesn't help me keep my job and bring in more work. I don't want to just help my patients; I want to be the one who makes their lives great! And I want to be the one they hire!

Have you ever seen a spy movie with secret agents? And the secret agent is in one place in the world driving a fast car, and in the next scene, they are jumping from a plane, and in the next scene they are dancing in a formal gown or tuxedo? Caregivers are like secret agents, too.

Okay, so we may not be doing the same things as a secret agent, yet like a secret agent, our jobs constantly change. And how we handle these daily changes not only tells our employer whom to hire, it also makes the client feel respected.

One day we are on diaper patrol, the next day we are stopping a breathing machine from waking up our patient. The next we are clipping finger nails, and the next going to get the mail. We are like secret agents; we don't know where or what we are going to be doing the next hour, the next day or the next week!

We could be cooking, reading out loud, finding lost keys or hearing aids, singing a bible hymn, buying new batteries, picking up prescriptions, etc. We are the secret agents that no one knows about except to those in the business. We save lives every day!

In helping you to do your job better, I have put together a list of the most helpful ideas that I know. I have put these ideas into a list of ten rules.

These rules are very important, and set up a basic operating system that we can work with. Once you learn these simple rules, your job and the odds of you keeping your job and getting additional work will increase dramatically. These rules took me many years to learn, and they will save you years worth of mistakes, and loss of unnecessary income. Here they are in the order presented in the book:

Rule 1: Respect the Boss

Rule 2: Respect the Boss's Medical Team

Rule 3: Respect the Boss's Behavior

Rule 4: Respect the Boss's Limits

Rule 5: Respect the Boss's Privacy

Rule 6: Respect the Boss's Property

Rule 7: Respect the Boss's Trust

Rule 8: Respect the Job you do for the Boss

Rule 9: Respect your Boss by Increasing your Worth

Rule 10: Respect the Laws of the Boss's Land

Bonus Rule: Respect the Boss's Finances

Each patient you take care of will have you interpreting these rules differently, yet respect is the most important element no matter who you are taking care of.

When you begin with respect, beautiful things can happen. For instance, we allow our patients to grow and change as time goes by. In many ways we become like parents who adapt to our children's needs as they grow, and as our client's age and change, we change with them. It is a beautiful journey.

Please remember; as the older population ages, there will be more business for you than you can personally handle. And once people recognize you as a hard working and respectful caregiver, you will be recommended and become part of people's families.

Successful Caregiver Tip*: It is a wonderful gift of respect to know the details about what your patient's wishes are in case they get sick, pass away or in case of another emergency. This information is collectively written down in what is called an Advanced Directive. Some of you will need to know this information, others will not. Each case is different. Included in an Advanced Directive are such things as:*

- *Call orders. Who to call in case of emergency and in what order. And hopefully a complete phone number list.*
- *What your patient's last wishes are for comfort and care. Is there a DNR order in place (a Do Not Resuscitate order), or certain requests for comfort measures such as oxygen or blood transfusions? Do they wish to stay at home or be taken to a hospital? Etc. Very important.*
- *Also knowing and having access to a complete list of medications is a wise idea.*
- *And being safe and having a complete and separate list of phone numbers to call in case of emergency or need. Make sure to include all medical team, family, and fellow workers. This list should be available to all staff, yet out of sight.*

Your work and value as a lifesaver are important!

It really is all about respect. If you have ever wondered why the good caregivers stay busy, and the rest only complain, then this book is for you and these rules will help you to understand why. Okay, let's go to work!

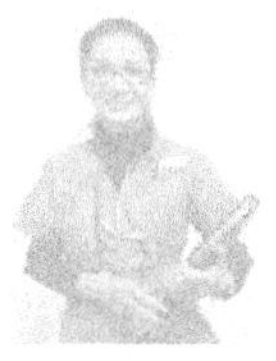

RULE 1: RESPECT THE BOSS

Overview:

"The Boss is always the boss, even if you are the one who takes care of everything. We are not saying that they are in charge of everything, for if they were, they wouldn't need you. We are saying that if they are self aware, it is a good idea to let them 'think' they are the boss, and maintain this respect in all conversations with the Boss throughout the day. This ultimate respect will impress others, and they will seek you out to take care of them when the time comes."

Explanation:

We all want to feel good about ourselves and a **Successful Caregiver** knows how to do make his or her patients feel good. When we can make the people we serve feel good by respecting them, they will want us around. No one wants to be around someone who doesn't like us, or make an effort. You must make this effort because your future employment depends on it.

Growing older is the most difficult thing most of us will ever do; it will be the challenge of our lives. The discipline required to do the simplest of things could make a busy college student shudder. What used to be easy now requires work, and what used to be done without effort, now requires assistance. And who wants someone to help us?

This is not an easy task for anyone who can employ a caregiver. Think about it, if you worked hard for many years, saving all your money, being the boss of our own life, would you appreciate some young person, a caregiver, coming into your home and telling you what to do?

For example, most of us like to dress ourselves. How would you feel if you couldn't? Most of us enjoy the privacy of using the bathroom on our own. How would you feel if you couldn't? What kind of mood would you be in if you couldn't perform the simplest of tasks? Tasks that make you feel independent and strong? What then? You would do what most older adults do; desperately try to control something…

It is very respectful to take care of all the little things that your boss needs doing, yet ask them what they would like to do. In other words, be respectful enough to give them some control back. Let them make decisions if they are able to safely. Give them this respect as their world becomes smaller.

Successful Caregiver Tip*: There is an old saying that says 'To the world you are just one person. Yet to one person, you may be the world.' This is naturally true when we are thinking about our children. We understand the need of the child to build confidence and security within a parent/child relationship. We understand this is healthy.*

The same idea holds true for older adults. Yet the difference is that the older adult becomes more dependent as times goes on, and we need to give them support during this transition. As their world becomes smaller, you become like the parent who has the power to say 'yes' and 'no'.

This is very difficult for an adult who more than likely has been in charge of their lives for many years, and you must respect this. You must respect that the truth is, they would rather be younger and healthier, and not have you there. Please respect them enough to let them make decisions and let them keep a perception of freedom when everything in life is taking that freedom away. They do not need to be reminded of how powerless they are; respect them enough to make them feel like they have control and you will be rewarded with continued work. Your future jobs depend on this first Rule of Respect.

Examples:

Good Examples:

Here are some simple ideas to show your boss respect:

- Call them sir or ma'am.
- Let them think they are smarter than you, and tell them in little ways.
- The Boss is never your friend; the Boss is the boss! Be friendly with them, yet remember you are there to work. Friendship is earned through a respect of the relationship.
- Compliment your boss; tell them they are beautiful or handsome. (Be careful with the men if you are a woman- set your boundaries if they get frisky!)
- Take care of little things without being asked.
- A wonderful empowering trick is to offer them several choices. Would you like this, this, or that for lunch? Milk or coffee? Ice cream or cake? Choices make us feel like we are in charge, and we appreciate a person who is gracious enough to give us choices. We feel respected. (continued)

- (continued) Retirement homes and hospitals use this empowering choice daily. Try it out. However, if a person is embarrassed or in a bad mood, just get the job done, because too many choices can become irritating. You have to respect them enough to find the balance.

Bad Examples:

Here are some examples of what not to do and say. Saying things like this do not show any respect and limit a person's choices making them feel powerless. Do not say these things:

- "Why are you asking? You can't have anymore ice cream- you know the rules."
- "No, I told you we're having chicken, or no dinner!"
- "Where are you going? You have to sit down! What's the matter with you?"
- "No, you don't know what you're talking about!"
- "You don't remember anything!"
- "Don't you lie to me!"
- "No, you're wrong- that's not what I said you old bat, what I said was…"

Don't talk back negatively, whether in English or another language. We can all detect when someone is upset even when we don't understand their language. And nothing is more infuriating than someone talking about us, right in front of us, in a language we don't understand. (Have you ever had your nails done in a salon where everyone is speaking a language you don't understand, and yet you know they're talking about you?) When upset, be smart and quiet in that moment. Don't talk back, even when they're wrong.

This is about doing the job, not your pride. *As I like to say, "No pride-chicken!" Pride will cause you to lose your job in the end. When an older patient is dying, remember it is one of the most difficult journeys we take; they have more reasons to be upset than you do. Your job is to save their lives, and sometimes they will be unkind. Let it go, and do your job. Treat them like family- good family!*

Certainly stand up for yourself, politely if they overstep their boundaries, and each adult has their own way they need to be dealt with. Whichever way this needs to be done, do so with politeness and respect. Think about how strong it looks when the President of the United States, or other politicians stay calm when heckled by a reporter. Please do the same.

You must learn to stay in charge of who you are. Don't be like those crazy people on YouTube who get angry and look absurd reacting in an out-of-control tone.

Being a **Successful Caregiver** is not a reality TV show! Be bigger than that. You are the President of your own caregiving company. You're the boss of you.

Successful Caregiver Tip*: Do not put up with abuse. There are many kinds of abuse in this business and you do not deserve to put up with any of it. Please learn the difference between the anger and confusion that an advanced Alzheimer's patient may project toward you, and the difference between real abuses of someone just being mean. Thankfully, most of you as licensed caregivers will have access to resources that can help.*

If you need to walk away from an abusive patient, then walk away. You will discover the kind of patients you enjoy as time goes by and those that are right for you. There are also family members, medical staff and conservators that make life difficult. If you must leave, it is always a good idea to put your resignation into writing to protect yourself.

Sometimes the case just isn't right for you, and there is no wrong doing. Different cases are for different people. I specialize in terminal end of life cases, yet close friends of mine like their bosses to be younger and more active. Don't be afraid to discover what works and doesn't work and you find your way!

Conclusion:

Respecting the Boss is really about being able to consistently look at your situation as if you are the boss, and adjusting your actions accordingly. Being a **Successful Caregiver** requires attention to the smallest details, and each patient will have a learning curve that you will adjust to as time goes by.

In other words, you will learn how to take better care of your boss as time goes on. For instance, is your boss in a good mood? Are they unclear as to who they are today, as to who you are today? Did they sleep well? Did they eat well? Have they gone to the bathroom? Etc. Paying attention to the details and adjusting is very respectful.

In the same way that good manners makes for better dealings with everyone, and prevents many problems, respecting the boss works in the same way. When you respect the boss from the very first day, you will do things that make you stronger and empower both yourself and your clients. Do this, and your business will be in a position to grow!

Simple Summary:

Rule 1: Respect the Boss

- The Boss is always the Boss, even when you're the boss.
- Find ways to help them, without making them feel bad; empower them.
- If possible, offer choices.
- Be polite by referring to them with a respectful title.
- Compliment them and treat them like loved family members.
- Respect is a practiced art, and we all need reminding daily.

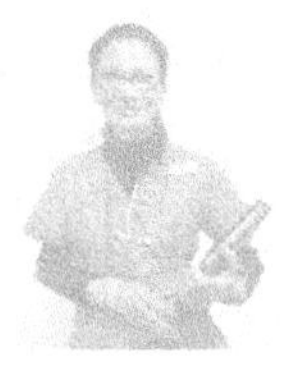

RULE 2: RESPECT THE BOSS'S MEDICAL TEAM

Overview:

"One of the most important parts of being a caregiver is respecting the medical team, because YOU ARE PART OF THE TEAM. You have information and knowledge about the Boss's daily activities that the medical team needs to make informed decisions. You must learn the confidence to share this information, respect what each specialist does, and assist where appropriate."

Explanation:

The Boss at some point in time will have a medical team that helps them. Sometimes this team of people will know each other, sometimes they will not. Sometimes they will need your communication to let them know what is going on, and you should always be prepared to provide helpful information about the Boss. So how do we do this?

First off, understand that the Boss's medical team is like a wheel, with each professional being a cog on that wheel. In the center of this wheel is the person or advocate in charge of the case, and this person (who could be family, social worker, conservator, etc.) will be in charge of contacting the medical team and often takes care of billing and insurance.

As a caregiver, our job is to help the person in the center of the wheel do their job. We do this by providing up to date information that the advocate can give to the medical team, or sometimes we will present it ourselves. How we present this information is important and can help save a life. Let's examine what you need to observe, record, and then share and or report about. There are two primary areas that provide the facts you can share with the medical team:

What you see and observe each day.

What you record and write down in a log each day.

Each of these two areas is important.

The first point, your observations, is concerned with the needed details of what happened that day with the Boss. Did they fall? Were they dizzy? What did they eat? How were they feeling, etc. This information is needed by the medical team to treat immediate needs the Boss may have.

The second point, a written record, is concerned with sharing what you've written so that the medical team can look for patterns in the Boss's behaviors and abilities. This information is needed to establish base lines of existing protocols to see if they are working or not. This information will be used by the medical team for medications, food concerns, sleep patterns, long term cognitive observations, etc.

If you keep track of both of these areas, you will be best prepared to help and assist the medical team if needed. And the best way to do this is:

Keep a written record of the Boss's daily activities.

- You can use a spiral notebook or three ring binder.

- Keep track and write down when the Boss woke up, napped, and went to bed.

- What time they took their medications, and what they took (do this even if you are in a retirement campus situation or a hospital) and why.

- Did they exercise? What did they do and for how long? Did they go out? Get their hair cut? Shower today? Brush their teeth? Keep track of bathroom habits, etc. Each case is different; please make your own charts.

For those of you on night shifts, it is very important that you keep a written record. This is because sometimes the Boss won't remember how many times they get up each night, nor what their sleeping patterns are, or won't take their pills, and your information could be very important, and could even save a life!

Bad Examples:

Perhaps the worst thing a caregiver can do is to not be respectful about being an important part of the medical team. Here is what NOT TO DO:

When asked about what the patient ate, or how they slept, or what their toilet habits were try not to say, "I don't know."

I DON'T KNOW' says to the medical professional:

- You don't know your job.
- You don't pay attention.
- You're just a baby sitter who doesn't care.
- You didn't care enough to ask.
- You didn't care enough to communicate.
- You're not professional.
- You're uneducated.
- And, "We should really get someone else in here who knows what they're doing."

Please understand that saying 'I don't know', when you do not know is not a bad thing, but saying you don't know because you have not been paying attention and doing your job says you're wasting everyone's time.

Therefore bringing up what you do know about the Boss says you are a professional, even if you're unable to answer a specific question. I have known caregivers to lose jobs because they didn't pay attention, or were dishonest and lied about what they knew. Worse, I've watched caregivers being interviewed and watched them lose the job because they couldn't answer specific questions about how they take care of the Boss and work with the medical team.

There is no way to fake being a caregiver who cares enough for the patient; your actions and your words will show who you are. I realize that what I am suggesting is extra work, yet this will mean you keeping your job and having future work. And that is a good thing!

Successful Caregiver Tip: *In a circumstance that requires your Boss be in the hospital, especially for an extended time period, many times you will need to go to the hospital with them and then stay. There is one main point you need to know about the laws and regulations within the hospital: When you are at home with the Boss, you are a caregiver. When you are in the hospital you are now called a sitter and <u>no longer a caregiver</u>.*

In a hospital situation, many Bosses like to have their own personal caregivers come with them, and for good reason. Sometimes the staff is overloaded with work and may be late with meals, or therapy sessions, etc, and a caregiver can provide wonderful advocate services on behalf of the Boss– yet this is done as a sitter and not a caregiver.

- *A sitter stays with the Boss, and provides company.*

- *A sitter does NOT administer medications, provide therapy, adjust machines, etc.*

- *A sitter is simply there for the sake of the Boss's comfort.*

The reasons for this aren't because you don't know what you're doing. Many of you are more than qualified than the hospital staff to care of your Boss. The reason is that insurance and health laws prevent you from working as a medical professional in that environment. Even if your licensing is the same as employees of a facility– you are <u>not an employee</u>.

However, when working with the Boss in the hospital, you will discover many areas that you can fit yourself into without breaking any laws. You can help with the food, you can help the nurses and staff to change diapers or slide a patient up in a bed. Bring messages from family, etc. Eventually, if the hospital staff trusts you, they will gladly accept your help– just wait until you're asked!

Examples:

Good Examples:

There are many things a caregiver can do when assisting the medical team. Here are some ideas:

- While you are never in charge of medications, you should be able to provide a simple report to the nurse/pharmacist/or person in charge as to how the patient is doing if asked. (If there is a concern about medications, ***report it immediately***.)

- For example, if a patient doesn't remember not liking a medication, you could say, "He/She has complained about this medication, or this new brand, etc." Or-

- "This pill seems to upset His/Her stomach". Or- "He/She keeps falling asleep or is very confused when they take this pill."

- And while it is not your job to administer medications, if you do have a concern, please report it immediately to the doctor or medical professional and write it down.

- Learn how to take blood pressure, especially if in a private home.

- Make sure your patient drinks enough water, as dehydration is a very common cause of hospitalization, and then keeping a written record of what they drink is very professional.

- If a patient has bed sores, keeping track of when you move them, when they are changed and any other facts will give you much credibility with the medical professionals around you.

- Please note: If you work with another caregiver who isn't doing their job, and you come into situations where you suspect a person has fallen or is bruised, whether or not this person is your Boss, you must protect yourself. Please take a picture with your cell phone to protect yourself and keep a written record, a private one if necessary. And certainly, if you suspect abuse of any kind, in most cities within the United States, you are mandated to report this abuse to the state or city. Be cautious about reporting abuse within a facility without proof. And it is usually safer to report this kind of activity directly to the state Ombudsman, where the reporting is confidential.

- There are people within the health care industry who will be very nice to your face, and turn around and blame you for things that are their fault. The best way to protect yourself is to get to know the staff and family that works with the patient. For some of you, myself included, this was difficult. My natural inclination is to be quiet and do my job. Yet as the years have gone by, I have discovered that not only do I do a better job by communicating with those around me, I also protect myself.

Successful Caregiver Tip: *Think ahead about what your Boss will need. This is what good medical professionals will do; they consider their patient, what they need, and make the necessary recommendations. And since you are a part of the team, learn to look at what your Boss needs for today and tomorrow.*

The best way this is done, as in any business environment, isn't to try a hundred things randomly. It is rather to ask a better question directly related to your Boss. The best question asked is:

***What does my Boss need me to do today,
that will help their mind, body, and spirit,
not only today, but for the future as well?***

Once this question is asked, you can be better prepared to be a **Successful Caregiver***. Here are some ideas.*

For Example:

- *Do you think your Boss needs exercise? Can you take them for a walk, or ride a floor exercise bike, or play simple games of movement in a chair with them? Check with the doctor or medical staff.*
- *Do you think your Boss would benefit from group activities such as Bingo, or playing Bridge, or from reading?*
- *Do you think your Boss (for a lady) might enjoy some nail polish, or lipstick. (Or for a man) Or would he enjoy wearing his nice shoes and dressing up? Of course all of us like to have someone comb/brush our hair, and make a fuss over us.*

- *Do you think your Boss would enjoy some music, and having you sing with them? Try it out. If you're in a retirement home, are there computers that your Boss can use to play brain games?*

Ideas like this can help a patient live a happy life. And there is no end to how you can help. Please respect your position enough to go the extra mile!

Simple Summary:

Rule 2: Respect the Boss's Medical Team

- A caregiver is a part of the Medical Team.

- You provide valuable information to assist the team.

- You provide information in two areas:
  ~ Through your observations
  ~ Through your written reports

- Your job demands that you pay attention and remember in case of need.

- When in the hospital you are no longer a caregiver, but a sitter. Please respect the hospital environment.

- Doing extra things to make your Boss comfortable and communicating these kind gestures will give your employers confidence in you and future work recommendations.

- Ignoring your patient, and then having to say, "I don't know" because you don't- will eventually cause you to be terminated. Know your Boss!

- Think ahead about what your Boss needs and plan activities that will be good for them in the long run. Plan events and activities for each day, week, and month.

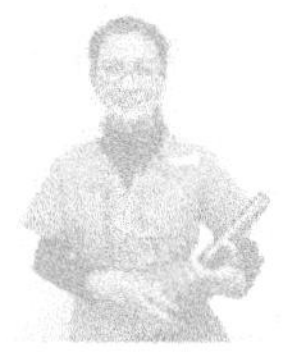

RULE 3:
RESPECT THE BOSS'S BEHAVIOR

Overview:

"The Boss's behavior is to be respected, even if it is different. (Certainly we are assuming nothing bad or illegal is happening to you and that your work conditions are safe.) Sometimes, the Boss is just odd or has developed interesting or different habits. They are entitled to these habits. Please work with them with love and without judgment. When others see this patience and kindness, they will ask you to work for them, too!"

Explanation:

Life can be difficult physically for anyone, and as we get older it can become even more so. Now we know this; we are trained caregivers, but most older adults have not considered this. Most older adults go kicking and fighting into old age and the need for help.

Most have not prepared for the physical ailments that old age can bring, and many times we as caregivers will find ourselves re-educating patients in the simplest of behaviors and skills. In return, many older adults are not easy to deal with. And the list of what older adults can be like ranges from complaining and depression to irritability and tantrums.

Yet though this can be difficult, we must learn to respect their behavior. We know more about what they are going to go through than they do, and part of our job is to be a guide for them on this their last journey.

Successful Caregiver Tip: *As a general rule, women are easier to deal with than men. I don't say this for everyone, and I have been blessed to have had long term cases with both men and women, I will just say in the aging process, usually, women are easier to deal with.*

In fact, many families will hire caregivers for their fathers, while usually if there is an older woman or mother, she will hire the people herself. Though each case is different and unique, women usually are better prepared to slow down and deal with things.

Men usually will push themselves to do more, and get hurt in the process. And men like to think that ignoring the problem will fix the problem. In the over used cliché of "A man goes into his cave to fix his problems", is the perfect metaphor for older men. Here are some funny examples of how men handle things:

"I have Heart issues? Just wait, I'll be okay..."

"I don't feel that bad… Just wait, I'll be okay..."

"So I fell down, and something popped, and now I'm bleeding everywhere- don't worry, I will be okay. Let's just wait a while…"

Men tend to get... more like men the older they get. Please, keep your eye on your men, and while you must respect their behavior, call 911 if you need to or get someone to help you!

Here is something important to consider as well: Sometimes older patients will become angry at their situation, and then blame you because you're the closest person to them. You have no right to argue with an elderly patient. There are two simple rules in business and you should memorize them:

1. The Customer is always right.

2. If you have any problems, go back and read the first rule again.

Now this is not to say that your patient isn't wrong and that they need to stop. Some elderly people can be very cruel and even vicious. If this happens to you, document in writing what happened, and then walk away from these types of people, and/or seek professional help. Do not put up with abuse, nor try to justify it in anyway. Protect yourself and leave the case. And remember, when you are confident enough to say 'no' to a bully, they will usually back down.

Please do not hesitate to call the local ombudsman and file a complaint if you have been abused or treated unfairly. However, we must not get upset and engage with a patient who is not doing mentally well; their anger belongs to them and not you. Let them be angry without getting involved in their anger. In the same way a smart parent knows how to let a child be a child, so too should you let an upset older adult be an upset older adult. (Assuming that is the safe choice to make!)

Therefore if you are safe and you have an older adult who has a few odd behaviors, let them go if it's okay and not harmful. In addition, while respecting these behaviors, please keep these behaviors confidential. (More on this point later) We must learn to *respect* our patient.

Examples:

Good Examples:

Here are some common behaviors, and while you will try to keep your Boss busy with productive behaviors, you may experience these.

- The older adult who wants to get up early and get dressed for work, even though they don't work anymore. Then they spend the next two hours reminiscing, only to have fallen asleep in their chairs two hours later, and they do this every day... *Respect this.*

- The older adult who has to have the phone with them the entire day just in case one of their children call… *Respect this.*

- The older adult who has bowel troubles and blames the food he's eating that day for it, and then refuses to eat that food for the next two days, only to completely forget a week later, and eats it again, with no problems because the food wasn't the problem in the first place, and the entire time, blames you... *Not easy, but Respect this.*

Bad Examples:

Here are some examples of behaviors that, while you must respect the Boss's individuality and personality, you need to seek immediate help and assistance:

- The older adult who refuses to get up during the day to go to the bathroom, only to get up all night to pee… *Work on this one- get help.*

- The older adult who shouldn't drink or smoke but still does, and when you find them with cigarette butts and empty bottles, tells you that they didn't do it even though they did… *Work on this one- get help.*

- The older man who wants to put his hands all over any woman… *Work on this one- get help- DO NOT PUT UP WITH THIS ABUSE IN ANY FORM.*

- The older adult who doesn't want help in the bathroom, and then proceeds to make a huge mess… Or goes to the bathroom alone to make an even bigger mess! *Work on this one- get help.*

- Confusion and difficult behaviors that are beyond your knowledge or job description. Please get help and write everything down in a log book- this could save your job. Read the tip below…

Successful Caregiver Tip: *I once had a very difficult patient, who became abusive towards me. However, when I told the family about their father's behavior, he then said that I was abusing him! Thankfully, I had been documenting his behavior and I was able to show the family, and save my job. Medications were then adjusted, other caregivers brought in, and the situation turned out well. Yet without any proof of my innocence, I could have been held liable.*

Conclusion:

We must respect our client's behaviors and oddities that occur with age, yet as our examples clearly show, we must not allow behaviors that hurt anyone, meaning our patients and ourselves. And this can be a fine line.

For example, the older adult who is stuck in bed and dying, has reoccurring urinary tract infections, yet loves his sugar and wants his sweets. Obviously, sweets are not good for UTI's, but if a patient is dying, do you give them a dessert? These are all cases where common sense must be measured against medical advice and family wishes.

Get the help you need from the medical team if you deem it appropriate, and also seek the wisdom of older caregivers. There are many wonderful older caregivers who have been working for a long time that you can talk to and get general advice from. I say 'general advice' because you must not discuss private information about your patient to people outside the case. We will speak about this in a later chapter. Not only is it unethical, is also against the law. Therefore, ask other qualified caregiving professionals only general questions to help you take care of your patient better.

Simple Summary:

Rule 3: Respect the Boss's Behavior

- The Boss may have unusual behaviors; if they are safe, and no one is being hurt, nor are personal boundaries being exploited, then respect them. (Though please get assistance and advice if needed.)

- Balance out the effect of the behavior on the well being of the patient. If they feel better sitting close to a door, imagining someone is coming to see them, this may be better than having them sitting in front of the TV. (Seek help if need be.)

- Never point out the oddness of a patient's behavior to them personally. Please be supportive, kind and respectful. (Seek help if need be, especially if you are dealing with a difficult patient.)

- If a patient is being abusive toward you in anyway, please document this to protect yourself, and then seek professional help immediately. Do not stay in an abusive environment. You are a professional caregiver; you are important and valuable. Please protect yourself if need be.

- And finally, respecting behavior never means letting a person hurt themselves; it means finding the balance of what works for them in a safe way for everyone involved. This is not always easy to discover, but if you respect your Boss, you will find it.

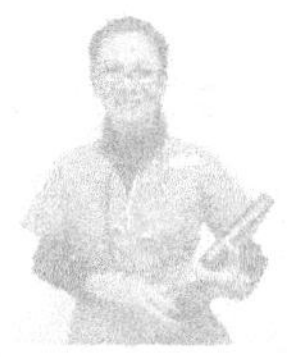

Rule 4: RESPECT THE BOSS'S LIMITS

Overview:

"Let the Boss have their limits and don't push them to do things they cannot do. When there are things they can do better, inspire rather than order. Remember: In any human interaction, limits are overcome with respect and inspiration. Though you must know how to be strong and give orders when necessary, respect how this is done. Inspire your patients to be better each day and always maintain a respect for how much they think they can do, versus what they can do. It is a great gift of respect to see people for who they think are, when they are not that person anymore. This respect will be your calling card."

Explanation:

Why are you reading this book? Who do you think you are? Why don't you just give up and quit now? You can't do this… *Imagine if I said that?*

Doesn't feel very good does it? Being told you can't do something hurts everyone. We all need to be told we can achieve our dreams now or in the future, and this doesn't change with age. In fact, my role in being the author of this book is to share with you facts and stories that will inspire you to do a better job. You want me, as the author of this book, to give you something- to teach you something and to INSPIRE you. Your Boss needs this, too.

If I do a good job as the author of this book, you will feel inspired, do a better job, find more work, earn more money, have a better life, etc. My job is to respect you and help you be a better caregiver. Your job as a caregiver is to respect the Boss so you can become a better caregiver for your Boss.

You must discover ways to empower your Boss to make them feel better about themselves. Sometimes this is as simple as going into the garden and looking at the flowers, or having them discuss their children or when they met their spouses. For some a little communication is all that's required, for others working on a craft activity is needed. And though each case is unique, every person will benefit from this additional love and respect.

Yes, you must know your Boss's limits, yet within those limits, you can make them feel proud about what they can do.

Successful Caregiver Tip: *I once heard a story about a dance teacher inspiring his students. A young male student approached the teacher. He was upset that the dance steps he was learning were the same dance steps everyone else was learning. And he felt he was a* *special dancer, and should therefore learn special steps. The teacher smiled and said, "It's not the dance steps that make a great dancer, it's how you dance them."*

As caregivers are we in charge of how we dance our dance, or do our job. Yes the steps (boundaries) are defined for us- but we can dance (work) with them anyway we like! If we have a chance to help motivate a relationship in a positive way, we can make our Boss proud to do the best dance steps (meaning their daily activities) that they can do today. Get them to enjoy the time they have left by respecting their limits, and then getting them to live and love what they CAN DO!

Examples:

Good Examples:

- Respecting limits can mean saying NO! Yet when you do say no, always offer another choice or two. Not as a bribe, but as a way to show them there are other options, and that you're not saying NO just to have control. In fact, many times the word NO from a patient can have a bigger psychological reason behind it, especially when they say no to things that they should want.

- Inspire them and you may just discover the real reason they say NO so much. You may turn a No into Yes! And certainly seek professional help if there

- (continued) are psychological issues and medical issues needing attention. Social workers are great for this kind of support, for they know the insurance laws and benefits a person is entitled to. Part of being a **Successful Caregiver** is building a good team of other professionals you can trust.)

Successful Caregiver Tip: *Family visits are exhausting. It is a simple fact that adults who have older parents think that their visits and outings are the best thing for mom and dad. Yet the truth is family outings can be tiring, and older adults usually won't say no to their kids, because they want to see them. This ends up getting your patient exhausted and then you have to deal with them when their adult children go home. It is perfectly okay to tell your patients children that their mom or dad is exhausted after a visit if appropriate; they need to know that these changes are normal, and you have to find the right time and circumstances with which to bring this up. Sometimes involving a social worker or nurse is good. A fitness trainer I knew used to say to my clients children, "Visit twice as often, stay half as long". Sometimes less can really be more.*

- Here's another great empowering tool: Cut their food into bite size pieces without them seeing you cut it up. In other words, cut it up before you give it to them if they have trouble cutting the food. If there are things you can do for them, without them seeing you do this, they can feel proud of who they are. Most of the time they will know that you're busy taking care of

- (continued) little things for them. No one needs to be reminded of what they can't do. Do the little things that make their life easier because you care. Let them have their Pride Chicken- not you!

Bad Examples:

- Doing things right in front of the patient because you're too busy to wait, and you've lost your patience! Never do this, and this can be hard. Remember your patient can feel what you feel...

- Reminding them that they can't do things because you're the one that has to do them, and how much extra work it is, is demeaning and abusive. Yes you have to be firm, but being mean as a way to communicate is *never appropriate*.

- Telling them in mean ways, "Hurry up. What's a' matter with you?" "Why can't you use your napkin- you're so messy!"

- "Don't you poop- if you do, I'm not changing your pants- you just wait!"

Comments like these are wrong and abusive. They can get you fired, and will not get you recommended for future work. Be nice, always, even when you need to be firm and strong. This is a skill **Successful Caregivers** never stop working on, especially with difficult cases.

Conclusion:

Inspiring someone takes work and skill, and is not always easy. There will be times when you are at your wits' end with a patient, and you still need to be respectful.

If you don't think you can do this, that is perfectly okay; however this can mean that this is NOT a business for you. And if this is true, then you need to move on because in this business, respectfulness is a way of life. Without it, you will lose your temper, lose your job, and develop a bad reputation. (And we all know those caregivers who should be doing something else... Don't become one of these!)

Successful Caregiver Tip*: Exercising with patients. Legally you are limited as to what you can and cannot do with a patient, yet there are always exceptions to the rules! Learn what you can and can't do, especially within a retirement campus. Retirement campuses may have staff and doctors who do not have the best interests of the patients in mind, and though you may be helping someone, you could get in trouble. Each situation has its rules, so check up to see what you can do. Making sure your patient gets out every day and exercises and/or goes to social gatherings is a great way to establish a solid bond of trust and caring between you and your patient. However, please check first.*

Simple Summary:

Rule 4: Respect the Boss's Limits

- Inspire your Boss even when you give the orders.
- Make a person feel like they have some control even when they don't.
- Like a dance step, respect what they can and can't do. And whatever they can do, do it with joy and fun, and you'll both enjoy the journey!
- If appropriate, get your patient out to do some kind of exercise and activity. Yet please confirm what the rules are before taking any actions.

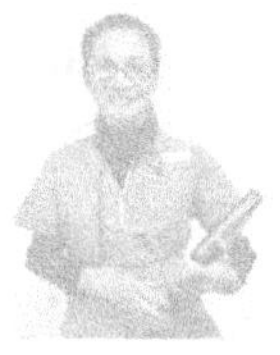

RULE 5: RESPECT THE BOSS'S PRIVACY

Overview:

"Give the Boss privacy in all ways; from gossip, from family, from friends, from nosey neighbors, from uninvolved medical staff and help, etc. Give them as much privacy as you can when showering, during toilet and changing duties. Give them the privacy of feeling taken care of when quietly combing their hair, applying lotion to their skin, and putting on their shoes. Keep the conversation light as if these private moments and tasks are getting done without your help, and you will help your patient keep their pride. Find ways to give them strength without showing it, and let them need you without them showing it. Sometimes just listening is the greatest gift of privacy and intimacy between people. This will make others want you to take care of them as well."

Explanation:

The Boss needs your help, and needs their privacy at the same time. Part of your job description is to assist the Boss with various things, and in so doing, you will be exposed to information that is private and confidential. The Boss needs you to keep to yourself their intimate moments of bathroom activities, night time activities, etc.

There is a great value in the world of business to be able to keep secrets, and those that gossip do not get the business.

Be aware too of the greatest threat to your future in finding work, and that is other gossiping caregivers and medical staff. Do not talk to these people who will ask you for details, and then share with you details about their patients. And if you must talk to them, let them do the talking and you will learn all about them. (Though you must keep your secrets to yourself, that isn't to say you shouldn't listen and learn from others- you will find out about many jobs this way- but be careful! The company you keep is also the pool you swim in!)

Successful Caregiver Tip: *We spoke about being a Secret Agent before. Imagine if you went to work for the government as a Secret Agent. How would they know how to trust you? You would be tested, and then receive a security clearance.* ***Successful Caregivers*** *give themselves their own security clearances. Gossiping is breaking your own security clearance! I have seen good people lose their jobs because they talked to everyone. Sometimes they were fired, but believe it or not, the biggest reason they lost their jobs was because the family and medical professionals wouldn't recommend them. You really are like a Secret Agent with a security clearance- the government that you work for is your Boss, and the penalty for gossiping and sharing secrets is the death of your job! You will lose in the end. Shhhhhhhhh...*

Examples:

There are a thousand things we could write and read together about what's not proper to share. If I were to offer a broad overview, it would be:

- **Never talk about your patient to anyone else not directly involved in the case**. There are laws in place that protect patients' rights, and if you gossip and share private information, you could be held liable for this violation.

Good Examples:

Someone may ask you:

"So Marta, I hear your lady keeps you up all night and smells really bad."

You reply with:

"My lady is just fine, and I can't say anything. Please ask the family."

Or, "My lady is just fine, and I don't remember anything."

Or, "Oh I'm so sorry, she is so private, I can't say anything or I will be fired."

Handle the situation as best you can and yet do so without saying anything about your client. If you get into the habit of gossiping, you won't make much money for long!

Bad Example:

A bad caregiver is asked:

"So I hear your lady keeps you up all night and smells really bad."

They reply with:

"Oh boy, when she BMs, it smells so bad, my eyes hurt…"

Or: "Oh yes, she's crazy, and she stinks, she won't shower, and I tried, but she won't listen, so fine, I let her smell- even her daughter can't stand her mother's smell."

Or anything that violates your patients or another's privacy! Become the keeper of the secrets!

So don't talk to:

- Neighbors and other nosy people
- Friends and family not directly involved
- Other caregivers
- Other staff members/nurses/medical personal not directly involved

Simply say to people who are too nosy, "Please speak to the family, or the medical person in charge of the case." Real medical professionals and other staff personal know they have no business speaking to you about the patient and are aware they are breaking protocol. They are breaking the law by asking you to discuss private information.

Do not get involved with people like this, or when they get fired, so will you. Worse yet, they will find a way to get you fired if someone suspects them. Be nice, be professional, yet maintain your distance.

If you want to keep your clients,
Keep your Client's Secrets!

Conclusion:

We all know those who gossip. They could be educated or uneducated- gossiping is a choice that people make. You must choose to make the right decision and keep your clients confidential information confidential, or suffer the loss of a job and a poor reputation. Gossiping in the end isn't worth it.

Simple Summary:

Rule 5: Respect the Boss's Privacy

- The Boss needs your help, and you need the job. You will learn things that are confidential, so keep them confidential- don't share them.

- Keeping the Boss's secrets is one of the highest forms of respect you can give.

- If someone isn't involved in the case, don't tell them anything private.

- DON'T GOSSIP! When others talk about you behind your back, let them; it will pass. Certainly protect yourself, but don't gossip in return.

Realize that as a truly hard worker, you will have to deal with lazy caregivers that don't want you to make them look bad, so often they will try to make you look bad. Don't get upset and cry and say, "They don't like me..." or, "Why are they saying bad things about me..." They own that negative behavior– you don't! No Pride Chicken- keep doing your work, have faith in the Lord, and it will all pass... Amen.

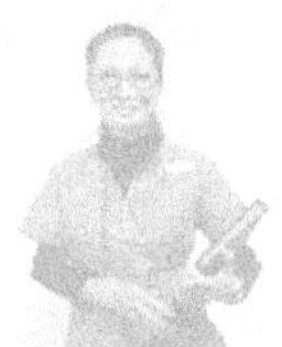

RULE 6: RESPECT THE BOSS'S PROPERTY

Overview:

"Respect the Boss's tangible items, such as personal property which does not belong to you. Try not to use anything in your patient's home or apartment if you can help it. Try not to use their phone for personal calls, and use your own sparingly. If you stay with a patient, bring your own pillow and food if appropriate. If you have a bathroom and shower in the patient's home, keep this room spotless- wipe out the shower, the wash basin, keep the hair off the floor, keep the toilet clean and neat- and do this every day. The goal is to make it look like you <u>do not live there</u>, even if you do. You are not a guest. You are not a friend. You are not family (even if they say you are.) You are a visitor who happens to also be an employee. Do these things as a matter of habit, and other families will want to hire you. Respect their property completely."

Explanation:

There is an old saying; "Familiarity breeds contempt." And in many cases it's very true. The phrase means that when we know someone or something very well, we can easily disrespect it and treat it poorly. Never feel this way about the Boss's property.

You must always realize you are a visitor. Their house or apartment is not a hotel, and their belongings are not yours in any way. Respect their property; what they have is not yours, even when they say it is.

Some of the contents within this chapter will pertain to those of you that will be live-in caregivers, and work 24 hour shifts regularly, and you will know this advice when you read it. However this advice is for every caregiver in any situation where personal property is dealt with.

> ***Successful Caregiver Tip**: If you keep personal belongings in your patients' home- make them look neat. A very simple way to make your belongings look good is to cover them with a blanket to keep them out of site. Always try to make things look tidy and simple.*
>
> *A wonderful way to make yourself look professional is to leave things on your bedside table or near you that make you look more professional. Ideas such as keeping a log book nearby where you are working or a bible or holy book near your bedside table, or a simple crossword puzzle book. The idea is to present you as professional and modest.*
>
> *If the family goes into your room and there are clothes on the floor, the bed isn't made, shoes and socks are*

lying around, a pizza box is in the corner, and you left the TV on, and the remote control is buried underneath 25 magazines and old makeup kits... then you can almost count on losing your job.

While you may be messy in your own home, as a caregiver be very tidy- no matter how messy your Boss is! (This includes clothes in the closet- keep them neat, minimal, and out of site if possible.)

Examples:

Good Examples:

- Keep the kitchen clean of any traces of your food; it's not your kitchen.
- Keep the toilet area clean and smelling good when you use it.
- Keep the closet usage to a minimum if you can, and keep it neat.
- Keep your socks and shoes kept out of sight.
- Keep your bed made and neat; you are the maid of your own hotel.
- Keep cups and plates out of sight in your room.
- Keep the volume of the TV down low, or better yet off altogether during duty; instead, watch TV with your patients- watching their shows, not yours.

Bad Example:

- Do not let trash overflow in your room and bathroom wastebaskets.
- Do not leave dirty laundry lying around.
- Do not spend your time on your cell phone. (Spending your work on your cell phone is stealing; pay attention to your Boss, not your phone! You are being paid to work, not play on your phone. This happens often, especially with younger caregivers who think no one will notice. Believe me, everyone notices. ***Stay off your Cell Phone, except minimally and privately.)***
- Do not take long hot showers in the Boss's house. You are not paying for the hot water; shower quickly.
- Do not use up all of your patient's personal effects, such as toilet paper, deodorant, toothpaste, food, spare change, socks, etc. Bring your own.

Conclusion:

Respecting the Boss's personal property is a wonderful calling card for future business. (And though we haven't mentioned it, it is also a great way to protect yourself against dishonest caregivers you may work with.) Use your own belongings as often as you can and keep everything tidy. In some cases, there may personal items from the Boss that you will need to use, especially if you're on duty, but the idea is to remember who they belong to and respect this.

***Successful Caregiver Tip**: When you put your own personal food into the refrigerator; keep it out of site– even if your Boss is not able to get up and look inside. Remember that other medical professionals, family members or those in charge of the patients' case will see inside the fridge at some point, so like with your personal belongings, be neat about your food.*

This also works well to protect your food. I have seen family members come over and eat their parents and my food because they felt they could take whatever their parents had! Some kids never grow up.

Protect your food and your job by finding the most hidden spot in the refrigerator. And if you need to use a cupboard to store additional foods, do so with a cupboard that is out of the way from the main area, and try not to use the Boss's pantry as a place to store things. Again; it should look like you don't live there.

Simple Summary:

Rule 6: Respect the Boss's Property

- The Boss's property is not yours and you should never take it for granted.
- What doesn't belong to you should be respected and if possible not used at all.
- Make it look like you do not live in the Boss's house; hide your personal property, and/or keep it in your room out of sight and stored neatly.
- Keep everything neat, in all areas, at all times.

God gives you what you want,
when you respect
what He has given to others.

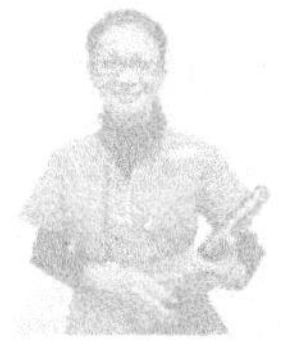

RULE 7: RESPECT THE BOSS'S TRUST

Overview:

"Respecting the Boss's trust is more than just understanding the need for privacy: The trust the Boss gives you is that of taking care of their life. This is more than a job; it is a holy mission of the highest order. In the same way that a child offers us their hand when they need help, so, too, our Boss is offering their hand to us and we must honor this request. When the Boss hires you, they trust you with their life."

Explanation:

Your patients (your Boss's) hire you to assist them with perhaps the most difficult and final part of their lives. This is not an easy task for anyone. Let me ask you, who would you hire to save your life each day? Who would this person or team be that you would allow to come into your home, perform life saving skills, and whom would you trust with this? Would you feel safe, knowing that the smallest thing that goes wrong with that caregiver's performance on the job could mean your death? Would you pay them more? Would you rather not let them into your home?

This becomes a very difficult question when you take it personally. Who would you let in? A stranger? Someone from an agency? Someone who could come in, steal from you, and put your life at risk, all in the course of one eight hour shift? The trust your Boss puts in you is a very big deal; it is life and death to them.

For we the caregivers, a job is a job. For a Boss, it's life and death. You are given a chance to honor this trust when you are hired as a caregiver, therefore you must realize that your job is very important, even if this job is only a transition for you, you still must give your Boss complete respect. You are like a parent responsible for a child, who now happens to be much older than you!

With the inherent difficulties in trusting another to this degree, it is not uncommon for the Boss to mistrust you in the beginning. This is because trust should be earned, not given. So don't feel bad if they are skeptical of your motives, and let your patients learn to trust you bit by bit. If done with patience and respect, many caregivers experience deep love for their long term patients, and their patients love them like family in return. A firm commitment of respect can open up your future in ways you can't imagine.

Therefore it is a wise idea to understand what the Boss, his family, and you are thinking during a job interview. When you understand the needs of each person involved, you have a powerful asset at your disposal. Here are some examples of what each person is thinking during the hiring process!

Examples:

Examples of what the Boss is thinking when they hire a Caregiver:

“Hiring is easy, trusting is hard!”

“Are they going to steal from me?”

“Will they be there when I need them?”

“What if I fall?”

“What if I need to get something from the store?”

“Are they going to take things away from me like my children do?”

“What about my medications?”

“What if I lose something?”

“Will they get mad at me, or argue with me?”

“Oh Lord, I don’t remember their name…”

Examples of what the Family is thinking when they hire a Caregiver:

“Hiring is easy, trusting is hard!”

"Are they going to steal from my parents?"

"Will they be there when my parents need them?"

"What if they can't stop my mom or dad from falling?"

"What if I need them to get something from the store?"

"Are they going to let my parents get away with things?"

"Are they going to stop my mom and dad from calling me 20 times a day?"

"When I hire them, will I finally have some peace and time for my family?"

"Will I finally be able to relax and catch up with my own work?"

"Oh Lord, I hope I spell their name right on their check…"

Examples of what You are thinking when you are hired as a Caregiver:

"I hope they like me…"

"I hope they don't fire me…"

"I hope I can get my paychecks…"

"I hope I can pay the rent…"

"I hope I can find time to speak to my children…"

"I hope I get Christmas off…"

"I hope they sleep at night…"

As you can see, three different perspectives for one patient, and as a caregiver you must know these perspectives so you can deal with them properly. Please deal with each party in the patient/caregiving relationship with the respect that each person deserves. You must learn to look at life through another's eyes to be great at your job, and though no one can ever completely understand another, it is the effort to be empathetic, and not just sympathetic that will set you apart. Another great word is 'compassion' for each of the different people on the case.

So you will have a relationship with the patient, that will be different from the relationship with the family, and from the medical staff, and your agency, etc. Remember that you are the glue and strength that allows the Boss to function with the world successfully and you must therefore deal with each person in your Boss's life accordingly. It's not always easy and you will always be learning- who said being a Caregiver is boring? Never! Slow sometimes, but never boring!

Conclusion:

As you can see, each person has their own perspective when it comes to trust based on what that persons role is. Yet as Caregivers our understanding must encompass all the people involved in the case, and this includes medical personal, and social workers.

Successful Caregiver Tip: *I once heard a story about a famous Hollywood actress who was worried that she wasn't performing her part very well. So one day, after shooting, she went up to the Camera Man and asked:*

"Did I do my part well today?"

~The Camera Man replied, "Yes, you looked wonderful!"

She asked the Light Man, "Did I do my part well today?"

~The Light Man said, "Yes, you were lit beautifully!"

And on it went...

~The Makeup woman said her skin looked flawless!

~The Hair person said her hair was perfect!

~The Director said he was so happy they got the shot!

The moral to the story is that people don't see you for you; they see you in the context of what they're doing. ***Successful Caregivers*** *see the people they work with, in the context of what they do. They talk to the family in one way, the nurse another way, the Boss yet another. And they do this without lying or breaking trust. At the end of the day, the respect and care of the patient is what will keep you working and have others recommend you.*

Our job is one of the most sacred jobs in the world and it is an honor to help a person experience another day of God's world each day. Do not take the trust handed to you lightly; respect it. Dying is hard and the trust you earn with your patient is everything.

Simple Summary:

Rule 7: Respect the Boss's Trust

- Trust is earned, not given.
- You are here to save a life; teach them to trust you.
- Respect that different people on the case will have different opinions and needs, and you should deal with each person based on their personal involvement within the case.
- Form trusting relationships with each person, keep confidences, and of course never gossip!
- Be honest with everyone, say less, listen more, and respect, respect, respect!

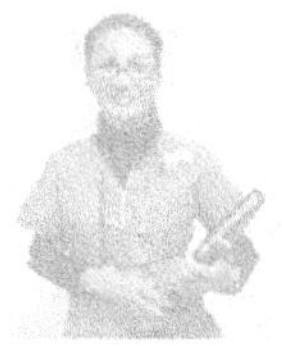

RULE 8: RESPECT THE JOB YOU DO FOR THE BOSS

Overview:
"The Boss will ultimately treat you the way you treat yourself, so love yourself and respect that you are doing one of the greatest jobs in the world. Very few people can successfully do what we do. Very few. There will be those who look down upon you when you do your work. Smile and know that only weak people look down upon others, and that the same person judging you today, could be asking for your help tomorrow; even if they couldn't give you respect, give it to yourself. And then watch your business grow!"

Explanation:

I once read a book by a psychologist that said, "When you wear a mental sign that says "KICK ME", eventually everyone will kick you!"

One of the simple truths in life is that others treat us the way we treat ourselves. Good or bad, right or wrong. How we feel about ourselves is the guide to others on how we want to be treated. This includes your boss.

This is important because many older adults will not have the ability to be diplomatic when you feel bad about your life. And I respectfully will share that I understand that many of you have pain and hurt deep inside that has become a part of you; I had to work very hard to bring my children to the United States, and help them become legal citizens. This pain will never leave me, even though it is past. There were many sleepless nights worrying about my sons– yet I respected the Boss and my job enough to keep this to myself.

Ultimately, no matter what your pain, you must have respect for the work that you do while on the job. How you think about what you do is important. Have you ever heard the quote, "Imagination is everything"? It's true. How you think (imagine the world to be) is how you will act toward it, and how you act will bring a reply from life in kind. As the quote says, "As a man thinketh in his heart, so is he."

We have all met the shy girl who grows up and becomes beautiful, or the young man who grows up to be a real hero. And we have all seen what true confidence can do for a person. We must develop confidence in our work, regardless of what others say.

We must realize that our actions and decisions make lives better, and save lives as well. Be proud of who you are. From making sure schedules are followed- from showering to making sure our boss goes to the bathroom, the list is endless. These are life-giving and life saving actions and you must learn to respect them.

Like a mechanic who fixes the car so it is safe, to the plumber who fixes the pipes for running water, we caregivers provide actions that sustain life.

***Successful Caregiver Tip**: We have discussed that one of the best referrals you can have is from family and friends who are familiar with your work. When you respect the job from deep inside, people will see this conviction and recommend you.*

Have you ever had to deal with someone who didn't like their job? It's difficult isn't it? We have little respect for a person who hates their job and who doesn't like serving us. We all want to be treated nicely from this person. We enjoy those that enjoy their jobs, and we want to be taken care of by someone who cares. There is nothing worse than dealing with someone who doesn't care. We will never recommend them, so please don't be that person: Respect your job and the work you do, and your business will grow!

Examples:

Here are some ideas about how to think in successful ways. I have divided these thought ideas into two categories; **Successful Caregivers** and Poor Caregivers and what each would think. And we are going to define that the **Successful Caregivers** are the ones that think the good thoughts, while the Poor Caregivers think the bad thoughts.

Good and Bad Examples:

- Poor Caregivers think: I am only a caregiver, I am not that important to these people…
- Successful Caregivers think: I am blessed to be a caregiver. God has me here for a reason, and it is important, and I will serve as best I can. I respect my job!

- Poor Caregivers think: Caregivers are only servants, and the family doesn't care about us or our job…
- Successful Caregivers think: It doesn't matter what the family thinks, and even though that is hard sometimes, I provide certainty to my Boss and my family. I respect my job!

- Poor Caregivers think: I can never connect with my Boss because they don't like me very much...
- Successful Caregivers think: I can connect with my Bosses by caring about them more than their opinion about me. I am here to serve, and I am getting paid. God is great!

- Poor Caregivers think: This is a boring job. It's the same thing every day, and it's driving me crazy…
- Successful Caregivers think: This job may lack the variety I need, so I will explore other options that are more fulfilling for me. In the meantime, I have a job to do and a life to save!

***Successful Caregiver Tip**: And a quick word on how others treat themselves: How others treat themselves is how they treat us. And how we treat ourselves is how we treat them. Who we are comes out in the subtlest of ways- we really can't hide intense pain and anger. This is why I believe daily spiritual reading is important. For me, remembering God and his promises through reading gives me the faith to respect my job, my time with my patients, and the time I miss doing other things. For others this spirituality is found in planning goals and getting excited about the future. This is important because many of us will find ourselves feeling down when our Boss is down, and that's not fair to the Boss! Find something to inspire you every day, whatever gives you faith in life, then watch your business grow.*

Conclusion:

While this chapter sounds simple, it is not. Learning to respect the job and paying attention to how you express yourself professionally is constant work. We are social creatures by nature, and it's very easy to get off track in an environment where there are negative people around. Remember in a world of pain and people dying, you are the shining light they need. Please say a prayer each day, have faith in God, and respect that you are in the right place to make a big difference. If you want the respect you deserve, try giving it to yourself first!

And certainly, don't mix with negative people. Though you may have to work with them, you do not have to adopt their points of views and/or habits. Respect the job enough to mix with those who have the same goals in mind as you do!

Simple Summary:

Rule 8: Respect the Job You Do for the Boss

- Respect starts inside first; pay attention to your thoughts about your work and keep it positive.

- Every thought makes a difference; use healthy imagination.

- How you treat yourself inside is eventually how the Boss will treat you outside.

- Find faith in spirituality (however you define it) every day.

Respecting your job and the work you do
will get you referrals!

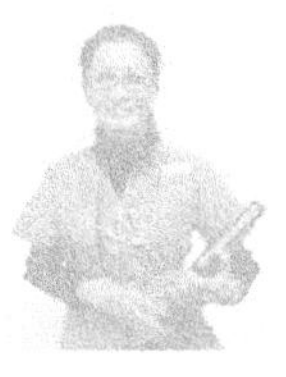

RULE 9: RESPECT YOUR BOSS BY INCREASING YOUR WORTH

Overview:

"The Boss will have other caregivers approach them looking for work, and they may offer their services at a cheaper price than you. There is only one successful way in business to counter this eventuality and that is to increase your worth.

We increase our worth by not only knowing how valuable we are based on our skills, but also through learning and educating ourselves in new methods of care. When we know more, our value to the Boss increases, and as we learn to do our job better, the Boss has more reasons to want us to continue to work. If we only do the same thing month after month, and do not increase our worth to the Boss, we are not respecting our Boss and could lose our job to another.

Therefore increase your worth and knowledge every day. This will fill you with confidence, which also has the effect of other Bosses wishing you would work for them. Your formal schooling is only the beginning of your education."

Explanation:

Knowing how much we are worth professionally can be broken down into two main areas:

- *The first is knowing what your skills are, assigning them a value, and adding them up. This will addressed in Part 1 of this Chapter.*

- *The second is deciding which areas of additional education you should pursue. And this will be addressed in Part 2.*

Part 1 Knowing your skills and their value.

So how much are you worth per hour? I don't mean the simple hourly rate that you know other caregivers are already paid; I mean how much you think your work is worth per hour. How much would you pay yourself if you were the Boss?

For some of us this is a very difficult question to answer objectively, as we may have had our sense of monetary worth damaged in childhood. Some of us feel that money is bad. Some of us feel like we do not deserve money, or any blessings. Yet I would ask you to please rethink this: You are very valuable, and there is a monetary value within our society for your skills. Please do the following exercise outlined in this chapter's **Successful Caregiver** Tip.

***Successful Caregiver Tip**: A wonderful exercise to do is to find out how much money you're worth per hour. When I ask most people what their personal financial hourly rate is, they usually tell me they are worth whatever they are being paid, and that they wish they were getting more money! With this blind approach to your true value, you will never be paid what you're worth. I am not suggesting you be greedy and ask for something you don't deserve, I am suggesting that if you have the skills, you should be paid accordingly.*

Take out a piece of ruled paper and divide it into two columns. On the first line of the first column, write the word Caregiver. Next to that, on the same line, yet in the second column, write the hourly rate you get or should be getting. As an example:

Caregiver *$15.00 per hour*

Next under that, following in the same format, list other skills and their appropriate pay per hour. For example, do you know how to cook? How much does a cook with your skills get paid? $15.00 per hour? Put that underneath the Caregiver line, and so on. Do you know how to clean- add $10.00 per hour... Baby sitting? $10.00 per hour. Pet sitting? $10.00 per hour... Clothing repair? $10.00 per hour... Typing and word processing? $15.00 per hour... Speak and read more than one language? $35.00 per hour... Write as many things as you can.

Now we will ADD THEM together...

- *Caregiver* *$15.00 per hour*
- *Cook* *$15.00 per hour*
- *Cleaning* *$10.00 per hour*
- *Baby Sitting* *$10.00 per hour*
- *Pet Sitting* *$10.00 per hour*
- *Clothing Repair* *$10.00 per hour*
- *Type/Word Processing* *$15.00 per hour*
- *Language Translation* *$35.00 per hour*

TOTAL: ***$110.00per hour***

From this we can see that a person with these skills is worth, oh my GOODNESS! $110.00 per hour! And if you really do this exercise, I'll bet you could add other skills! Please do this exercise right now!

The point of this exercise is not that you'll get paid that much to be a caregiver per hour, the point is that when you know what you're worth per hour, people will treat you differently because you KNOW WHAT YOU'RE WORTH!!! You will walk with much more confidence, and others will see it. When you know what you're worth per hour, that confidence will help God help you in wonderful ways!

Part 2 Other areas of knowledge to know and pursue

There are many things we can do as caregivers to increase our worth to our Boss. We can:

- Earn additional certifications.
- Renew existing certifications.
- Learn to take blood pressure.
- When in a private home, assist the Boss with chores and planning.
- Pick up medications from a pharmacy if you drive for the Boss.
- Subscribe and read medical magazines and journals.
- Assist with food preparation, laundry, and cleaning if appropriate.
- And many other areas.

The big goal is to make you worth more money and value by consistently doing a better and better job each day. You should NEVER do the exact same job month to month; you should always try to find ways to do your job better- INCREASE YOUR WORTH.

For some of you that could mean reading medical books, having a better attitude, picking flowers with your client, taking more walks with them, believing in God more, etc. If you can anticipate the changes that your client will be going through, such as advanced cases of COPD, or neuropathy, or Parkinson's, Diabetes, etc, and you learn additional skills, that is providing an additional value.

Good Examples:

A skill I see many caregivers perform poorly is that of answering the phone. You should learn how to answer the phone politely and in a happy way. And once you have been given permission to answer the phone, you will need to be polite and learn to differentiate between the important calls and the sales calls. Here's an example of how to handle those sales calls that plague the older population:

"Hello?"
"Is this the Campbell residence?"
"Yes it is."
"May I speak to Mrs. Campbell please?"
"Who is calling please?"
"This is Ann from Roofers R Us."
"What is this regarding?"
"We are offering new roofs-"
"No thank you, have a nice day." Or "May I take a name and number please?"

The Boss will usually be able to tell you who they wish to talk or not talk to, and sometimes their families will as well. If I were to recommend a formula for answering the phone, I would offer the three step beginning used on the previous page. (And please be energetic and friendly!)

Say, "Hello?"
Ask if you need to, "Who is calling please?"
Again if appropriate, "What is this regarding?"

Bad Examples:

Here is how NOT to answer the phone:

"Hello?"
"Is this the Campbell residence?"
"Who is this?"
"May I speak to Mrs. Campbell please?"
"What you want?"
"This is Nancy from Roofers R Us."
"She in da bathroom now; you call later." Or…
"She an old lady; she don't want your roof." Or…
"She got no money to spend for you… She can't pay me if she pay you!" Or…The worst of all…
"Okay, hold on, I get her for you…"

Not very professional. Your patient should want you to answer the phone, because then they come to rely on you in a healthy way. And yes in theory, how you answer the phone is up to the Boss, however in real life, they won't tell you what to do. They will usually listen to how to you do this and then instruct you. Therefore be as professional in your phone etiquette as you can. Here are some other ideas about how to take care of the Boss:

- Go and get the mail if appropriate, or use getting mail as a reason to get them up to walk.

- If you are cooking, prepare special treats. And let them know that they are special– give them a

- (continued) special name or make them on a special day. Retirement homes do this very successfully.

- Remind them when their favorite TV shows are going to come on. This helps give them a schedule.

I learned this powerful idea from my older sister Mae, who also happens to be a **Successful Caregiver** and my mentor (*She is the best!)*. Many years ago, she used to make coffee for one of her patients each morning.

Once she bought them a gift of Hawaiian coffee and they loved it, calling it 'Mae's Hawaiian Coffee'. And when the 'Hawaiian Coffee' ran out, she began using regular coffee instead. However, her patients still called it Mae's Hawaiian Coffee, even though everyone knew it was regular coffee! Her Bosses liked the name, and it stuck, and they asked for it every morning as a special treat! What my sister taught me is that when you give a normal food a special name, you make it a special food, and therefore something to look forward to.

So, I don't cook regular pancakes, I make "Fres's Special Pancakes". And because they have a special name, they taste better. Didn't special foods your mother made always taste better? So can your foods. Name your foods with special names and offer them as treats! This idea works on all of us, no matter the age!

All these ideas again go back to one main idea: We must increase the value our Bosses place in us regularly. We are here to make our patients live easier and increase their quality of life. This means we need to do whatever we can to earn our patients business and keep it. You may find your Boss bragging about you to their friends! Little things done daily add up to big things. And of course by increasing our worth, we are making ourselves indispensable.

***Successful Caregiver Tip**: Here are a few things Successful Caregivers do that Poor Caregivers do not:*

- ***Successful Caregivers** stay up and sleep very little on night shifts when their patient needs monitoring. Poor caregivers just sleep- sleep- sleep...*

- ***Successful Caregivers** ask to eat or go and get food when they're hungry if their clients and families forget to feed them. (Too many older adults and their families will not feed you nor pay attention to whether you eat or don't. It's just a simple truth- please always take with you light snacks or water whenever you go out for yourself so you don't lose all your energy. Granted sometimes, it is not right to say you're hungry, yet please do communicate when you are not being given basic meals.)*

- ***Successful Caregivers** constantly strive to improve how they do their job. New skills mean more money in the long run. (Sometimes adjusting and changing for others is the most selfish thing you can do!)*

Conclusion:

Respecting your worth and increasing your worth is very important. Knowing that you are more than just a caregiver in the strict definition of the word, and that you bring so much additional value to caring for others- and that those skills have a measurable financial value, is very empowering.

Interestingly enough, people who are abusive try to make those they abuse believe they have no value, so clearly knowing your own value, is perhaps one of the most valuable and proactive things you can do.

I'd like to say something about co-workers who are not nice. You may encounter them, and they may do mean things. Don't let them into your head and rob you of your inner peace. God will take care of them in His time. Forgive, forget, move on, and get the job done.

Simple Summary:

Rule 9: Respect Your Boss by Increasing your Worth

- Recognize that we are worth more than the single hourly rate for our job. Add up your values!
- Do little things each day to increase your worth.
- Learn new skills to increase your worth.
- Help and assist; make yourself indispensable.
- Don't let negative co-workers rob you of your inner peace.

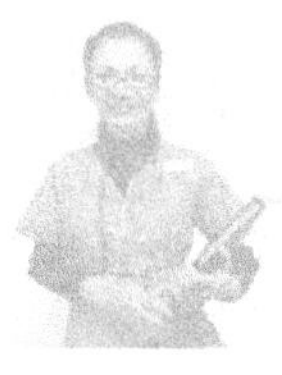

RULE 10: RESPECT THE LAWS OF THE BOSS'S LAND

Overview:

"The laws of country and city differ wherever we go, yet the truth behind them is usually the same: The laws came into effect through years of work involving many thousands of people. The laws exist to protect you and to give you a chance to become successful. They are not in place for you to seek ways to break them and not get caught. People that break the laws in small ways stay small. You can't grow into the person you want to be and be successful if you don't respect the laws. Please do."

Explanation:

Too many caregivers show up to a new country and never learn the laws. This is sad because countries like the United States are mixes of all races and there is place here for everyone if you can navigate the laws.

This is a country where your biggest dreams can come true, and I'd like to spend the rest of this chapter's information with good ideas that will help you run a better business. Within each of these suggestions is the implicit idea to embrace learning. Please read each section to understand the basics of it, then to learn how you can apply the knowledge, and what are the appropriate laws and licenses needed at a simple level.

Once you know the answers to these questions, you can then seek out the expertise of qualified professionals. (Please seek appropriate legal help, as my ideas are only my opinions, and not do not constitute legal advice in any way!)

Legalities

Setting up your business: Some of you will work for an agency, and others will work for yourselves. Whatever you do, learn the legalities of what you need to do. Get your appropriate licensing and stay current with the qualifications. Ideally, learn as much English as you can, for it will make life easier for business and communication with English speaking patients.

Get your own business cards

Business cards say to everyone that you know what you're doing. Hand them out to everyone you know, unless you're working with an agency and it is inappropriate. Purchasing and having business cards made up for you is easy and inexpensive in today's world. You can get them online, go into a printing shop, or have a friend help you. A basic package of 500 to 1000 cards is cheap enough, and there are always free card deals.

The basic information you want on your business card is your name and title of what it is you do, the name of your business, a great quote, your phone number and email. Putting a picture on the card or symbol is nice as well, and if you've been doing this for a while, mention how many years you've been in business.

Let's cover the most common mistake; making the letters too small to read for older eyes. Business cards for the caregiving industry should have writing on the cards that is a little bigger than normal so that older adults can see your name and phone number easily. Letter sizes (called Fonts) come in numerical sizes. The average business card font is size 8 or 9, and sometimes size 10. Ask your printer to go no smaller than size 12 and see if you can get your name and phone number in size 12 or 14. (The average book font is size 12, so it's really not that big, and this book is written in size 14 font. Easy to read isn't it?) This is a must so that older adults don't feel embarrassed when they read your card. Make your information easy to see; fewer words and bigger letters equal getting hired faster!

Next, put great quotes on the cards that promote what you do. Your card will sell people on your service. Here are some fun quotes; you can mix and match them, use one or make up your own: 'Licensed and Experienced'. '5 Years Experience' (or more/less). 'My family is your family'. 'Caring and affordable'. 'Experience you can trust'. Etc.

Now let's move on to phone numbers. Here is a common mistake: Caregivers who are just getting started using someone else's phone number and not their own. You should have your own phone number on the card and not someone else's. There was a time when you had to do this, but today with disposable phones in the store, everyone can get their own phone immediately.

Here's another reason why you need your own phone. I have worked with many Americans who try to reach a caregiver they are interested in hiring. However when they call the phone number they have, someone else answers the phone who may not speak English, or can't take a message, or is rude, or doesn't help at all, and the American patient just gives up, and you lose the job. You need to have your own phone number and some kind of message machine for your people to leave a message. If they can't get a hold of you and or leave a message for you, they will call someone else.

The next bit of information should be the name you go by. Put the same name on your business card that is on your bank account or driver's license. If you have a nickname, tell them later. You don't want the bank refusing to cash your checks because the name on the check and your bank account are different. Keep your names the same if you can.

A word about race and who gets the job.

A book like this would not do anyone a service if I didn't mention how race and culture play into getting recommended for jobs.

So often in the health industry, those within a certain race recommend others of the same race for jobs. This is not right. Recommending someone because they are the same race as you is racial prejudice and is wrong. Recommend someone because of how they do the job.

If you racially recommend someone, not only is that wrong, but if that person doesn't have the same respect and care for patients that you do, your reputation will be ruined. Remember, anytime you recommend a fellow professional to another Boss, they will assume you're recommending someone like you, and when that person turns out to be not like you, your hard earned reputation is now on the line, and your customers friends will not trust your recommendations anymore.

Let the small people fight about race and practice prejudice. Be bigger than this; we are all the same in God's eyes. If you're going to recommend someone to get the job, do so because of how they do the job, not their skin color or place of birth. And if members of your culture dislike you because of that, bless them and move on. They were not your friends in the first place!

A Word about getting your papers.

This is a special section for those who are working in the United States illegally. There are millions of undocumented workers here in the U.S. Though I am not qualified to speak about this, I am exposed to it and here is how I would summarize what I do know.

Get your papers and get legal. Though you may not know how to do it now, and it may seem like it is impossible, it can be done. Many caregivers live in fear of being deported every day of their lives. Many have families that they raise here and establish lives- even buying homes. All this can be taken away from you overnight if you do not become legal and get your papers as soon as you can.

Though this subject is beyond the scope of this book, and I cannot give out legal advice, don't think you're safe without papers; you are not. And hundreds of thousands are deported every year; do what you have to do to survive, but get legal, start paying taxes, and stop hiding as soon as you can. Have hope and pray- miracles happen.

If you don't have papers, please be nice to everyone you work with. I have seen workers with papers call Immigration on workers without papers because they were not nice. No legal immigrant in the U.S. who has worked hard, is going to let an illegal person who is mean, steal a job from them. Most people support good people. No one supports a mean person for long.

Conclusion:

Learning the finer points of business and law in whichever country you live in is one of the smartest things you can do. Learn all you can, as soon as you can!

Simple Summary:

Rule 10: Respect the Laws of the Boss's Land

- Learn the laws of going into business for yourself.
- Get easy to read business cards in large print for older adults eyes.
- Get your own phone number; one that you can keep.
- Be above racial prejudice; only recommend the best workers.
- Become a legal worker or resident, and get your papers as quickly as you can.

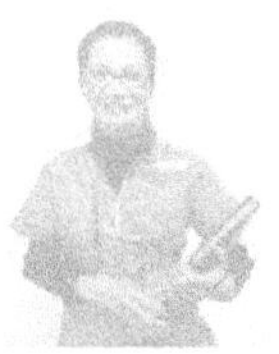

BONUS CHAPTER AND CONCLUSION

BONUS CHAPTER: RESPECT THE BOSS'S FINANCES

Overview:

"We must have a respect for the finances that belong to the Boss. The Boss's money and belongings belong to them. What they have is theirs, and not ours. You may hear other caregivers tell stories of receiving gifts of money or assets from the Boss, and some of these characters will try and find ways to take from the Boss.

There are very strict laws in place to prevent this abuse from happening. Respect what the Lord has given them, and He will give even more to you. It is better to give than receive. This sense of abundance will cause your business to grow."

Explanation:

The Boss's money (and/or) belongings, belong to them and our job is to take care of them, and that means we also protect their assets in small ways:

- We respect the Boss's money when we tell them the truth about how many hours we worked.
- We respect the Boss's money when we provide receipts for purchases and write things down to protect both our Boss and ourselves.
- We respect the Boss's property when we care for it and keep our eye on it.
- We respect the Boss's belongings when we put things away, or return items, or help them find things.

We must treat our Boss's belongings with respect by protecting them as best we can within the parameters of our job. For most of you, this does not require much of an explanation, yet there are those caregivers whose goal is to find a rich patient to take care of and do everything they can do to get in the person's will or to have them give them money.

While I understand the dream of finding a wealthy person that loves your work, seldom is the case in real life. More often than not, many older adults have difficulty paying us, and we need to respect the fact that if they run out of money, we will lose our jobs. This is why part of our job is to make sure our Boss's money and belongings are protected.

It is heartbreaking to hear fellow Caregivers bragging about how they tricked an older client into including them in their will, or into giving them money. What is most sad is that I believe there is no shortage of money in the world, and God will give us what we wish for if we follow His plan. Caregivers who work with older patients just to be included in their wills are the poorest of Caregivers. They believe in lack and their lives will reflect this.

In the United States there are Elder Abuse Laws in place to prevent caregivers from abusing older adults, because sadly in years gone by, many older adults were taken advantage of.

My advice to you is to stay out of the money situation all together. And protect yourself in every way possible. One of the best ways to protect yourself is to keep a log book of daily activities, monies spent (keeping all receipts), etc. There is an old saying in the medical field, and that is this, "If it wasn't written down, it didn't happen". Protect yourself!

So if an older client wants to offer you something or include you in a will, please check with your agency or at the very least, consult an attorney to protect yourself.

Remember, the Boss's money belongs to them!

> ***Successful Caregiver Tip***: *Be fair with your billing practices; don't over-charge or you will lose in the end. I know of one caregiver who was taking care of a friend's patient while she was on vacation. He was an older man who was very kind. He expected the new caregiver to be fair with him, and told her, "When you come and visit me in the hospital, I will be happy to pay for your expenses." Well, she was not fair with him. She only saw him for 7 days, for 8 hours a day, and charged him over $2000.00 dollars! Among the absurd things she charged him for: She charged him $20.00 each way for gas, $40.00 for two meals each day, and he was so happy she brought him flowers each day, until he found out she charged him $60.00 a day for flowers! He paid her just to get her away from him, and I never recommended her again. Don't steal the Boss's money; you will lose in the end. (And if you recommend someone, please make sure they understand the rules and how to be fair. Don't assume they will be fair, because many people are not.)*

Examples:

One of the things that happen to caregivers that are treated as family, is that they are offered material things. Sometimes this is a real offer out of love and kindness, and other times, the patient isn't thinking clearly. Here are some ideas as to how to handle this:

Good Examples: (Funny)

- "No Sir, you can't give me your house, it's for your daughters!"
- "I don't need a new car Sir- you need to keep your money! I need a rocket!"
- "What? I have more money that you Mamm, I don't need money, I am a multi-millionaire. I need happiness! You can buy me some of that!"

Bad Examples: (Not funny, and yet ALL true…)

- "I don't have any change for you. You got your food, and that's it!"
- "Oh, my son is having a hard time, and he needs money for his surgery… I don't have enough money to pay for it- can you give me some?"
- "I hope one day, I could have a house like your house… Oh yes, I would live here forever if you gave me your house…"
- "My friend, her boss is very, very nice; he put her in his will. That's what good bosses do."
- "My car is broken down, and it needs to be fixed…"

- "My family needs money back home, and I send them everything I have… Can you help me?"

Conclusion:

Our job is to protect our Boss. Being honest is the best policy in keeping a job and building a successful business, and that means respect their finances.

> ***Successful Caregiver Tip:*** *Some older patients become confused and will offer you money. They will offer you cars and even homes. This is a double-edged sword. Sometimes family members will say you stole from their parents, even if you're in the will, and will file elder abuse charges against you. Protect yourself by speaking to someone who understands the law. The best rule is to never accept gifts, and stay out of financial concerns.*
>
> *** If you are given-*** *cash to buy something, bring back a receipt and change. (The purchase price and your change must add up.)*
>
> *** Keep a log book-*** *of purchases if necessary. (I know of a case where the son of an older woman was stealing her petty cash, and blamed the caregiver. She would have been fired if she had not kept accurate records to prove her innocence.)*
>
> *** If you are offered-*** *tangible items such as furniture or clothes, etc., check with family members first so*

you are not accused of stealing later. (Some caregivers have a bad reputation, not because they have stolen anything, but because they never communicated they were given a gift, at the time it was given, so later on it was assumed they were stealing.)

*** Family members have been known to steal-** from their parents and siblings, and you could end up being in the middle of it. Please protect yourself legally if you can, and keep a written record of anything you can to protect yourself.*

You don't ever need to bring up anything about money or stealing. Your Boss will have already heard stories about theft. More than likely, the Boss's friends will have had or heard of bad caregivers who have stolen from their friends, and you may address any concerns openly within the context of a conversation. Protect yourself ahead of time, and then do the right thing.

***Successful Caregiver Tip:** You are there to help the Boss, and they are not your friend. Keep this idea in your mind when working. While you may end up becoming friends as time goes by, when you are working, you are a worker, never a friend. It is your job to be friendly, as if you're a friend, without expecting that friendship in return from the Boss- no matter how much of a friend they really are.*

There is an old saying, "The Rich Man doesn't need any more friends..." Be a fantastic worker and be friendly, and you may end up with a lifelong friend. Keep the two ideas separate or you could lose your job.

Simple Summary:

Bonus Chapter: Financial Respect for the Boss

- The Bosses' money belongs to them and not you.
- Be fair with your billing and keep a written record.
- Keep receipts and always bring back change.
- Do not ask for money from the Boss.
- Be aware of dishonest family members.
- Do not accept gifts from the Boss as a general rule. Yet if appropriate, please seek legal advice.

Respecting the Boss's money is important and says a lot about the caregiver. You will hear stories about caregivers being given large amounts of money or material possessions, and these stories usually are not true. However some Boss's are able to give presents to the staff that has helped them, and when this is done properly and legally, it is a wonderful gift. Yet let these gifts come in His good time. Please focus on doing your job, and everything else will be a blessing.

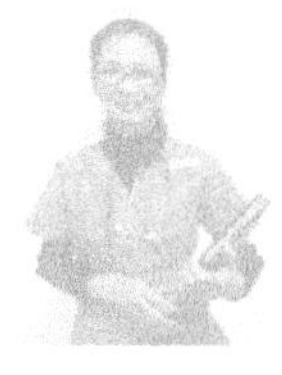

CONCLUSION

Thank you for reading this book. We have covered at lot of material in our short time together, and these Rules of Respect will give you the skills that can make you a **Successful Caregiver**. Let's repeat our rules in conclusion:

Rule 1: Respect the Boss

Rule 2: Respect the Boss's Medical Team

Rule 3: Respect the Boss's Behavior

Rule 4: Respect the Boss's Limits

Rule 5: Respect the Boss's Privacy

Rule 6: Respect the Boss's Property

Rule 7: Respect the Boss's Trust

Rule 8: Respect the Job you do for the Boss

Rule 9: Respect your Boss by Increasing your Worth

Rule 10: Respect the Laws of the Boss's Land

Bonus Chapter: Financial Respect for the Boss

These rules, if followed through with action will change your life. They will:

Increase your business in wonderful ways.

Make others want to be like you and recommend you.

And most important of all: You will earn the respect you deserve!

God Bless you. Thank you so much. Please contact me via email if I may be of any help. All emails that are appropriate will be answered. Please believe in your dreams. Our industry is the greatest industry in the world. We are the glue that holds the medical industry and the patients together. **We are Caregivers**; we are strong, we are successful, we are needed, and we are loved. I wish you great success, love, faithfulness, and peace.

Thank you for reading my book; I am very humbled to have shared this journey with you. God Bless you.

Fres D. Jacobo

You may reach Fres via email at:

- FresJacobo@outlook.com
- Facebook at: How To Be A Successful Caregiver
- On the World Wide Web at: **HowToBeASuccessfulCaregiver.com**

All appropriate emails will be answered.

This book may be used in the classroom with written permission. Contact email as above for releases.

Thank you. Please give this book to another who needs it and may your work be blessed! Salamat!

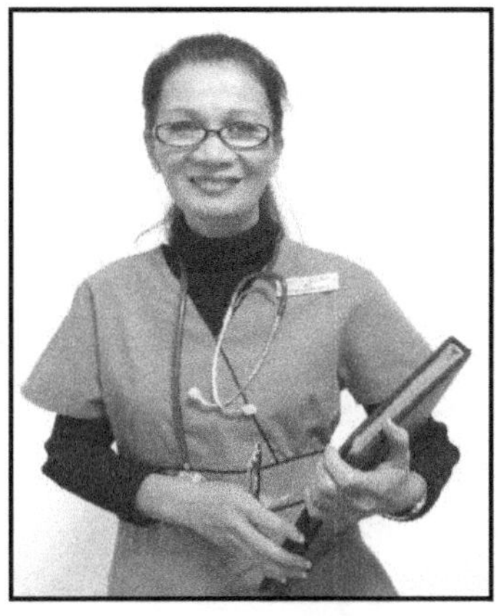